Mirthful
Memoirs
of a
Male Nurse

Vince Migliore

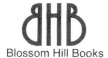

Blossom Hill Books

Title ID 3483550

Title: **Mirthful Memoirs of a Male Nurse**

Description: *Mirthful Memoirs of a Male Nurse* is an enjoyable peek into the nursing profession from a man's perspective.

ISBN is 1453818332
EAN-13 is 9781453818336
Primary Category: Medical, Nursing

Country of Publication: United States
Language: English
Search Keywords: nursing, male nurse, career
Author: Vince Migliore
Blossom Hill Books
113 Sombrero Way
Folsom, California 95630 USA
Reorder: https://www.createspace.com/3483550
First Edition, September 2010
Revised, April, 2011

Names have been changed to protect patient privacy.

Contents

It is a kingly act to assist the fallen.
- Mother Teresa

MOTIVATION

I want my life to have value. I want to know that what I'm doing has a direct and visible benefit to people.

I recently shook the strong, calloused hand of the grower at the farmer's market. He plants. He tends his crops. He sells it to the folks who eat it. I like that. It's a direct link to people. Simple yet powerful.

Sure, every job has value. Every service, every product does some good, somehow. Even paying taxes helps somebody somewhere. But, maybe I'm not that deep. I don't want to be three steps removed from the feedback. I want to see the smile on their faces.

Something in the medical field sounds perfect. People are sick. You help them. You see them go home healed. That's got to be good. The better you do your job, the quicker they are made whole. Yes, I like the medical field. It's a science and a service.

I've always been drawn to electrical instruments. Maybe an electro-cardiogram program would be the ticket. Maybe an X-ray technician.

I never thought I'd be a nurse.

"Your work is to discover your work and then with all your heart to give yourself to it."
- Buddha

DECISION TIME

I never thought I'd be a nurse. That's a lie.

I was 11 years old, playing games with my friends in the hot, humid streets of Brooklyn. We were pretending to be firemen. Then the game changed and I was a soldier. It was war time.

The game changed again.

"What do you want to be next?" my pal asked.

"I want . . ." My voice trailed off.

I was going to say I want to be a nurse and fix up those people who got shot in the war.

But nursing is for girls. I'll never be a nurse.
End of story.

* * *

Thirty years later, and I'm looking into
programs for Radiology Technician. I can't
seem to find the right school for training.

I ask around. I have some friends in the
medical profession. I keep hearing the same
idea. Become a nurse. Then you can go into
any specialty you like. You can work in
radiology or cardiology, or become an
Emergency Medical Technician.

All these ideas are just a flurry of snowflakes
whirling around in my head. There's not
enough mass yet to make a snowball.

* * *

I'm in the library, and I know they have the
course catalogs for the local colleges. It
turns out there is a junior college nearby
that has a 2-year nursing program. I look up
the class schedule. Wow! Today is the last
day to register.

It's decision time.

I drive over to the college, thinking it's
about time to act on this. There's a huge

room full of desks and fliers and people. I make my way to the nursing table. One of the people I ask for help happens to be an instructor for the nursing program.

"Have you taken the prerequisites? There are some courses you need to pass before you can enter the nursing program."

"Prerequisites?!" Oh, yeah. I did see something about that in the catalog.

"Yes. You know, you have to pass certain college level classes before you can be admitted. In fact, the nursing program is impacted. You have to compete with other students to be accepted. There's a waiting list."

"Sweet dreams and flying machines, in pieces on the ground."

"Well, I have a four-year college degree. In psychology." It was the only thing I could think of to defend myself. I could see the wheels turning in this woman's head. They were humming a harmonic tune. *Who does this bozo think he is? Waltzing in here thinking he's going to plow through the registration process.* But now, her gears were grinding, crunching, even starting to struggle in a different direction.

"Well, still, you would need to get permission from the program director, and I don't know where she . . . Oh, wait! There she is. Will you excuse me for a moment?"

She walks a few yards away to the Big Boss Lady. The director is the picture of efficiency; perfect hair, piercing eyes, and a posture that broadcasts authority. They are having an animated conversation, with glances in my direction. Good Lord, did I wear a clean shirt today? Is my fly open?

The gods are smiling on me today.

I'm IN!

"If you have to support yourself, you had bloody well better find some way that is going to be interesting."
- Katherine Hepburn

BACKGROUND NOISE

Ten days, two kids, 3000 miles. I'm driving across Utah on my way to California. Maybe my golden opportunity awaits me there. Brooklyn is already a vague memory.

Boxes and suitcases are lashed with bungee cords and rope across the top of the Plymouth. It's a wonder they don't blow away in chaos. Like my marriage. Tentative. Buffeted, but somehow holding together.

The words of the marriage counselor come back to me.

"I see you as frustrated. It's not your wife. You are searching for something. What is it? What have you always wanted to do?"

"I want to go to California."

* * *

They used to call it a midlife crisis. Now they have different terms for it.

It's not an event. It's an ongoing process, and it draws you in like some cosmic tractor beam. You find yourself in orbit around a foreign planet, wondering where you will land. All the while asking, *Why am I here?* A thinking man who examines his career will have to admit most of what he does is meaningless. If he's honest with himself he'll realize earning a living is generally a series of compromises, trading a decent paycheck against those undefined inner goals.

* * *

California has promise. Didn't they find gold out there?

I was confident in finding work. My resume included experience with the Federal Government, a security clearance, and a college degree. Surely there's adventure in California. I might even be able to transfer to the same federal job in California.

Eight days into the drive, I'm lounging in a motel room in Utah, watching television. President Reagan announces a hiring freeze on all federal government hiring. There goes my job! I have talent. I'll find something.

I was wrong. Six weeks in California and I still can't find work. *I'll just get ANYTHING until a real job comes along.* I looked at the classified ads in the newspaper. *Gas Station Attendant. Send resume to . . .* What! A resume for a gas station attendant? Words like recession and depression were in all the newspapers, haunting me.

* * *

In Brooklyn, one of my hobbies was astronomy. I was building a telescope in my basement. I loved science. I was grinding my own 8-inch lens. There's a lot of math and technology with this hobby. When I saw the ad for Optical Technician, I thought I'd give it a try.

Two years later, I'm grinding lenses for laser optics in a lab in Sunnyvale, California. I'm earning just above minimum wage. The marriage has unraveled, but I still have two kids to take care of, and I'm 3000 miles from my base. Now that cosmic tractor beam has me hurtling on a collision course with reality. I'm ready for a new career.

"The trained nurse has become one of the great blessings of humanity, taking a place beside the physician and the priest."
- William Osler

SCHOOL

Nursing school is fun. The uniforms lend an air of professionalism. The best part is the new vocabulary. A sphygmomanometer is a blood pressure cuff. You start sounding like a medical person when you talk. I have to buy specific supplies for some of the classes. The school bookstore has a section dedicated to nursing. I buy a stethoscope and a nurse's guide to pharmaceuticals.

The textbooks are massive and expensive. First, you look at the photographs. Next, you look at the chapter headings. I like to tackle a new subject that way. What are the major chapters? The text breaks it down into systems: the nervous system, the circulatory system, the digestive system. Finally, you actually start to learn some things.

I learned to fear every new malady that was described in class. *I might have that one. I definitely will die from this one. It runs in my family.*

* * *

My first day in a clinical setting is worrisome. Will I make it as a nurse? Nursing homes are often understaffed, so any attention a patient receives is highly appreciated, even if it's from a bumbling, naïve nursing student. My first contact was Nelly Dewe. She was 102. Our initial assignment was beds and baths. Make the bed, give the patient a bath, even if it's just a sponge bath. Nelly Dewe, a hundred and two. It had a nice ring to it.

After the basics, the instructors added other medical procedures. Vital signs, feedings, wound care. It worked out nicely. You actually do learn things. Finally they added the important skills, such as medications, tube feedings, catheters, and pre-op care. I stated to smile more often. *I can handle this!*

Even with months of preparation in a nursing home, the first day in an acute care hospital is a shock. Like a race car at the pitstop, everyone is busy. Fast-stepping nurses carry out the doctor's orders. Teams of experts apply machines and medications to every dent and bolt on the vehicle. It's a no-nonsense, near frantic mixture of medical procedures, medications, and human know-how. Above all, it's a team effort. Doctors work with the nurses. Dietary staff, housecleaning, respiratory care, and physical therapy are all intertwined with nursing care.

I was assigned to the cardiac surgery unit. The inter-shift summary of patient conditions was called simply the "report."

"Go to the 3:00 PM report."

"Sargeant, 15B. Cabbage times four on the tenth. Normal sinus. Elevated white count. Started PT today. Marshall, 16A. Mitral valve. Intermittent A-fib. He's now on a lido drip."

Sheesh! What the hell is that? I found out days later that it's simply shorthand for many of the things I was reading about in class.

Sargeant is the patient's name. Cabbage is short for a common operation, the coronary artery bypass graft, abbreviated CABG and pronounced "cabbage." Times four on the tenth means they replaced four vessels in the heart on the tenth of the month. Normal sinus means his heartbeat is regular. The white count is a blood test, and being elevated means there's a possibility of an infection developing. Mitral valve, in this case, means mitral heart valve replacement surgery. Intermittent A-fib indicates that post-op the upper chambers of his heart were irritable and beating too fast. The standard treatment for that is an IV drip with Lidocaine.

The report on each patient is followed by a series of numbers and initials, which are mostly vital signs and the results of blood tests.

Working in an acute care hospital is a quantum leap from the classroom. All the theory has to translate into physical action. Listen to the lung sounds. Take his pulse. Is he still having premature ventricular contractions? I have to record that in the nurses' notes. Better call his doctor too. We might have to increase his medications. It hits you: this is life-and-death material.

* * *

The two week rotation into the Emergency Room was a real education. Frankly, I felt inadequate. It's no place for novices. People show up with blood squirting out, in the middle of a heart attack, or with a finger in a jar, eager to get it sewn back on. It wasn't for me. I felt like I was in the way of the *real people* most of the time. Maybe after 10 years of experience I could go back there.

* * *

The Maternity Care rotation was a surprise to me. I never really could understand the allure so many nurses had for this specialty.

"It's a natural process. It's not a disease" they pointed out.

I was fortunate in coming from a large family with lots of younger siblings. Changing diapers was a no-brainer for me. I'd be burping one baby and changing another as my stunned classmates looked on. Aced that class.

* * *

Learning medications is the crucial part of nursing. Most meds can be taken orally, but some require injections.

There's needles, then there's the big gonzo "stabbers." I'm nauseous today, thinking I will have to use one of the bigger syringes, because it must be like getting jabbed with a pencil. Practicing on other student nurses, I found out that I hate giving injections even more than getting them. But I have to give my first pre-op shot today, and that means using a big needle with a thick gauge. Stacked in boxes in the nursing station, they range from the tiny, painless 25-gauge, ½-inch insulin needles all the way up to 14-gauge, 2-inch long monsters.

My instructor is cute. Miss Roselyn. She is years younger than I am, with a pleasant face, and teeth as white as her immaculate uniform. Alcohol swabs, vials of medicine, doctor's orders, and most of all the step-by-step instructions that are swirling in my head – they all come together in a nicely orchestrated dance, landing neatly on a metal tray. Miss Roselyn smiles her approval, but it's no comfort for me. This is going to hurt him. It's not only the length and thickness of the needle, but the volume of medicine; it stretches and breaks the muscle fibers.

She introduces me to the patient, explaining that it's my first pre-op shot, and gets his approval. This is for knee surgery. He's a college student, an athlete of some kind. Maybe it's track and field, because his muscular legs are noticeable beneath the flimsy hospital gown.

I ask him to roll over and I move the gown aside. There is one correct quadrant for the needle, and I swab it with an alcohol pad. One quick stab, and it's in, and he doesn't flinch – a good sign. A slight draw back on the plunger to make sure I'm not in an artery or vein, then I slowly inject the medicine.

Done. Mmm, not bad! I have him roll back to the sitting position. I want to get out of there as quickly as I can. I march out with the instructor.

"Well, how did I do?"

Suddenly, I'm horrified, because her face is red and sweaty, and she's not answering me!

"Oh, God! What did I do?"

"It's not you," she confesses, suddenly red-faced, "but when you brushed aside that gown, and I got a look at those luscious buns - - well, I couldn't see anything else! I'm sure you did OK."

* * *

I'm glad Miss Roselyn has a human side. I was just starting to hate her. She has a way of finding GLEs; Good Learning Experiences. I want to run the other way when I hear about a GLE. It's usually something horrible. Several GLEs have brought me to the brink of quitting the nursing program.

My first Good Learning Experience was collecting a stool specimen. It's repulsive enough to begin with, but this angry patient added several layers of difficulty. He had endured abdominal surgery, and the doctor wouldn't let him go home until he had his first bowel movement. It had been 5 days since the surgery; a long time to go with no doo-doo. But the stitches in the abdomen were still sore, and he just couldn't push too hard. There was a big fight between him and the staff. Finally, flushed with vein-popping anger, he vowed that he WAS going to take a crap if it killed him, and he WAS going to go home that day.

My instructor handed me a little container and a tiny wooden spoon. The kind of spoon you get when you open a Dixie cup of ice cream. *Disgusting!* Meanwhile, there's 20 minutes of wails and moans, grunts and screams coming from the man in the bathroom.

Bang! The door flies open.

"I'm outta here!" he shouts, as he starts packing his clothes into a suitcase.

But my torment is just beginning. I enter the bathroom, little wooden spoon in hand. There in the toilet is something you don't want to know about. Imagine a *Freddie Krueger* movie.

20

I think I'm "outta here" too. I toss the cup and the spoon on the floor and walk out. Maybe nursing isn't for me. As fate would have it, as soon as I left the room I almost crash into Miss Roselyn.

"Oh, there you are! Did you get the specimen?"

"Well, you know, I'm not sure that's going to happen."

* * *

Every now and then I see a complaint in the Letters-to-the-Editor section of the newspaper. Some money-oriented citizen is protesting that the nurses make too much money, and their union is a privileged special-interest group. If I ever find that letter-writer, I'm going to grab him by the neck and shove his face into that toilet and make HIM get the stool specimen. There is NO WAY that people will ever know the sacrifices that nurses make, and they are NEVER paid what they deserve. The doctors get all the glory. The health care plans get all the money. But, it's the nurses who are the real heroes.

* * *

Some Good Learning Experiences are actually good. Part of the schooling involves exposure to interesting medical tools. I was lucky enough to be admitted to a cardiac angiogram procedure. This is an amazing process to witness.

The doctor inserts a tube, a catheter, into the femoral artery in the groin, and threads it up the aorta to heart itself. With exquisite skill the doctor can position the catheter at the entrance to the coronary arteries, which branch off from the aorta and feed the heart muscle itself. When correctly positioned, the doctor injects a dye into the heart vessels. The result is a continuous X-ray image showing the beating heart with the black die now outlining all the snake-like networks of blood perfusion across the heart muscle. Suddenly there is a 3-dimensional image of that magnificent living organ. Of course the regular staff is trained to look for those bottlenecks in the angiogram which indicate a closed or blocked artery. But I was just amazed at the spectacle.

For me it was just short of a miracle; to see the minute detail of a real-time pulse was like being Superman with X-ray vision. Something odd happened. Like déjà vu or some psychic insight, the ill-defined intrusion of another reality broke across the operating room.

I could feel the presence of other beings around me; shamans and medicine men, healers and holy men, crowding around the monitor. They were watching too. They were smiling, nodding, and sending a clear wave-like message to me.

"Ah, maybe now you see. Finally, modern medicine can envision what we, the healers have known since ancient times."

"You send your child to the schoolmaster, but 'tis the schoolboys who educate him."
- Ralph Waldo Emerson

CLASSMATES

There are 22 students in my class. There are two students older than me; one woman and one man. There are only four men in the class. I like that. I like girls, and I like seeing pretty faces all around me.

I really didn't think much about nursing being a female occupation. I just wanted an interesting job with some potential for spiritual expression. I was recently divorced and having gone through a painful separation, romance was not on the agenda for me. Besides, you're dealing with life and death situations in this occupation. There is a lot of emotional turmoil among the families, and it's important that the nurses maintain a professional and supportive attitude.

One of the other guys in the class was a jolly, back-woods boy. Just two years younger than me, he was fresh from a 9-month sabbatical where he hiked from one end of the Appalachian Trail to other. I got a feeling he too was on some kind of path, searching for meaning in his life. The third guy was gay. Funny, but gays are generally outgoing and get along famously with the girls. This fellow, however, was moody and withdrawn. It seems he didn't want to talk to anyone of either gender, not even the instructors. The nurturing, warm-hearted mother hens on the staff tried to draw him out, but he resisted. Everyone was glad when he dropped out after the first semester.

The fourth fellow was the oddball. Heavy bearded with a sunken chest, his dark hair made him look dirty, even in his new white uniform. He just couldn't hack it in the classroom, and seemed to slink around during the lessons. It's a wonder the patients tolerated his secretive behavior. With the gay guy dropping out, I think the school wanted to retain the remaining three guys at any cost.

When we got to the study of the pharmaceuticals, Mr. Dark Eyes shined. He knew all the drugs, their street names, the uppers, the downers, the black market values, the effects, the side effects, the dosages and all their shapes and colors. It was the first module where he got an A grade.

* * *

The girls were a varied mix. Some were intellectual. Some were Mother Earth types, eager to heal the sick, rescue stray dogs, and save the planet. Many wanted to better their lot financially. A nursing degree enables you to move up a few levels, from the retail store clerk or secretary position to an enviable career.

The smart girls loved the science aspect of nursing, just like I did. There is so much about the human body that is amazing. It has regulatory systems, checks and balances, and an incredible depth of resiliency. Even when the body is abused, if you give it some rest and time to recuperate, it will bounce back nicely. There are complex processes involving hormones, proteins, electrolytes, and oxygen which keep us healthy. Learning can be fun.

Two girls were farmer's daughters. They were surprised when alcohol and tobacco were discussed in our drug abuse module. I was curious at their disdain for the hippie drugs, like weed and LSD.

"Country folks take that stuff seriously, you know. We grew up with drinking, but weed is like some liberal Yankee shit."

"Yeah, but you got Willie Nelson" I countered. "Isn't he a pot smoker?"

"Sure, but he's just considered odd by most country folk."

"Sex is the biggest nothing of all time."
- Andy Warhol

THAT SEX THING

Pretty close to 100% of American males have a sex fantasy about nurses. They think when they are admitted to the hospital that somehow, some gorgeous buxom blond is going to give them a hand-job.

Spoiler Alert! If you want to hang onto that fantasy, skip a few pages ahead. I am about to release of stream of urine all over that delusion.

Anyone who has worked for a living, anyone with social skills above that of Ted Kazinsky, knows that your co-workers become your friends. Many become like family. In the years I've worked with mostly female nurses, I've become close with a good

29

number of them. They have shared stories and confided in me their own fantasies and desires. Not once did I hear about some sexual interaction with a patient.

Imagine a barrel full of sand. Imagine taking one grain of sand out of the entire barrel. That is about the odds you have of being sexually serviced by a nurse. Imagine Tom Cruise, Brad Pitt, and Daniel Craig. Now look in the mirror. Imagine that face post-op with tubes coming out of every orifice. Yeah, you got a chance!

* * *

The truth about hospitals is that a very clear hierarchy is in place in the minds of everyone who works there. The hospital administrators have the power. The doctors have the respect and admiration. The nurses do the actual work. The patients are at the bottom of the pyramid. Even family and visitors are above the patients in the social pecking order.

That's not to say the patients are disrespected. It just means you're not going to get a date with a nurse. Maybe if you're a doctor you would have a chance.

* * *

I'm straight. There's never been a doubt in my mind about being a homosexual, just because I chose to enter nursing. It's a great choice for men. In fact I felt favored. I could pretty much go into any specialty I wanted to. I was thinking of working in the Emergency Room. I had one rotation there while it school. They need men there. There are often dangerous situations where the strength of a man is needed. People can be on drugs when admitted, or combative. Gang members have been known to follow a shooting victim into the ER to finish off the job. Lifting patients from a gurney to a hospital bed takes a lot of muscle.

* * *

You see a lot of nudity and become privy to some very personal information in the nursing field. You see people when they are most vulnerable. I often wondered if female nurses seeing naked men all the time, having to work on them, if that would somehow affect their desire for their partners. I asked about it. The universal response was *No*. For women, the attractiveness, the sexual desire and romance is mostly situational, a mood. They are still turned on by their husband or lover because of the social relationship, not so much by visual or physical triggers.

That was an eye-opener for me. Most guys can be turned on by a pair of water balloons or a blow-up party doll.

Actually, the distraction of physical attractiveness changed for me too. I was surrounded by women. Some were beautiful. But these are your working partners, and the work involves serious medical conditions. We are much more concerned with taking care of our patients than in fulfilling the roles you see on television dramas.

Some of the girls are alluring. I came to realize, however, that if they have no personality, no brains, or if they are incompetent on the job, then that is much more of a concern to me. Nursing takes dedication, focus, and knowledge. It's not a TV soap opera.

One time I had to provide on-the-job orientation to a new nurse. She was slender and was working part-time as a model. She was difficult as a new employee, reluctant to do the nasty stuff so common with nursing. There's a lot of ass-wiping tasks, both literal and figurative, in this profession. Like many nurses, myself included, there are times when you like the idea of being a nurse a lot better than actually working as one. She liked posing in her uniform, but not doing the work.

One day near the end of her orientation period one of the doctors commented, "Hey, who's that new nurse? She's quite a looker!"

"Spoiled" was all I could think of, but I bit my tongue and said, "Oh, that's Julie."

I was surprised that I had not really noticed how good-looking she was. I was more focused on getting her up to speed with the other, already professional grade nurses. I felt like maybe I had passed some kind of cosmic test; being able to see past appearances.

* * *

I had to look up some obscure medical question. I walked into the medical library at Stanford. With a white lab coat and a stethoscope around my neck everyone thinks I'm a doctor. That's a powerful advantage for a male nurse. It's not just for getting into the doctor's lounge or the library, but it also adds so much clout talking to family and patients. I'm often mistaken for a doctor. Sometimes I do not dispel the illusion, especially when the patient needs a lecture on taking care of himself.

* * *

I'm walking past the pharmacy. There is always a crowd there of people picking up their medications. As I pass by, a child is sick and starts puking on the floor. My instinctive reaction is to cover my nose from the smell and walk rapidly in the opposite direction. I look back, and a nurse from behind the counter is running out to the child and his mother, towels and water in hand, to help clean up the mess and comfort the young tyke.

I wonder, *How did I ever become a nurse?* I have none of those nurturing, embracing skills that seem to come naturally to women.

* * *

As a nurse, the body takes on a different meaning. Actually, it begins to lose the associations you've had with it previously. Nudity is no big thing.

I have a patient with an abdominal scar. I need to change the bandage and cleanse the open part of the wound. It extends right down to her pubic bone. As a nurse, I'm more concerned about keeping a clean sterile field and assessing the dimensions and conditions of the wound. I have to remember things so I can chart them accurately and report to the doctor when the procedure is done. I have a relatively new Nursing Assistant (NA) with me, and I have

34

to make sure she doesn't reach across the sterile area. I have to make sure I have all the right supplies: bandages, gloves, tape, hydrogen peroxide, alcohol swabs, scissors, and Q-tips. I have to unwrap the sterile packages in an orderly fashion and lay them out within reach.

"I'm not shy" the patient quips. "Modesty went out the window days ago."

She winks at me. I hadn't even thought about the nudity part, and I'm relieved that she is secure enough to joke about it. I guess this is the first time she's had a male nurse change her bandage.

* * *

A typical day involves nakedness. I have to examine people when they first come to the hospital. I have to observe and record all the physical details so we know what the patient came in with and what has happened since admission. Sometimes I have to insert urinary catheters or shave the pelvic area before surgery. The other nurses and I have worked out an arrangement. They will often trade with me; I will do the catheter insertions for the males who are too creepy for them or making sexual comments, and they will do the female caths for me.

* * *

I have an anorexia patient. She likes to have the window open when it's 90-plus degrees outside. She lays in bed totally nude. There's absolutely no danger of sexual arousal with a 70-pound body that looks like a Nazi camp survivor.

Still, we try to maintain at least a shred of privacy. We never let the family or visitors see patients uncovered. We always draw the curtains for privacy. As a male nurse I ask a female staff member to assist me during procedures that might be embarrassing.

Having a female co-worker accompany me not only provides some degree of professionalism for the procedure, but also provides for a witness against any charges of impropriety.

"The sick are healed when you let go all thoughts of sickness, and the dead arise when you let thoughts of life replace all thoughts you ever held of death."
- A Course in Miracles: Lesson 132

DEATH AND DYING

Death. It's a great black cloud that no one talks about. Except in nursing school.

They have well-researched programs on death. Nowadays both nurses and doctors are more aware, more enlightened about how to deal with it than they were a generation ago. There used to be a *conspiracy of silence*. Everyone agreed to pretend that the patient would be just fine. That stance denies them the opportunity to express their fears and feelings. Now, with the pioneering work of Elizabeth Kubler-Ross and others, the subject is no longer taboo. There is an entire movement to hospice care and natural transitions that has improved the care of dying people.

* * *

I was afraid of what I might find working with a dying person. It never panned out. The fear, that is. Death is most often painless and quiet. There was one devout Catholic woman who refused pain medications. She thought taking medications was against God's will. That was the only time in my many years of nursing that I witnessed a painful death.

The vast majority of deaths I witnessed were peaceful. No drama. The patient would often simply sleep more and more, wake less and less, and finally become comatose.

Sometimes an illness might entail discomfort. There are all kinds of ways to relieve pain. There are combinations of drugs, called cocktails, which are given to terminal patients to make their last days more comfortable. Now there are hospices and nursing homes that make the transition easier for everyone. Many hospice services will even provide home care, so the patient is in a familiar and supportive environment.

* * *

Blood and guts was another big fear. Again, there's not really a lot of that. Probably the worst experience is changing a bandage on a bad wound or infection. My first job was in the Cardiac Surgery unit at Stanford. There were a lot of open wounds, but they all healed well and closed up nicely.

One carotid artery surgery did not go well, and the wound became infected. The neck bandage had to be changed often. One optimistic doctor had posted a note on the wall.

```
"If the wound bursts, use
the hemostat to clamp off
the left carotid artery."
```

A huge, horse-sized hemostat in sterile packaging was taped to the wall beneath the sign. Yeah, that'll happen! No bursting blood vessels on my watch.

The only really gruesome experience was on the Emergency Room rotation. A patient had died from an automobile accident. Another nurse and I had to take him down to the morgue. When we lifted him from the ER gurney to the morgue station, the sheets were dripping blood in multiple pools. It was a repulsive experience, and very rare.

The other side of the coin is that you get used to things, especially if you see them often enough.

Chest tubes can be disgusting. After lung surgery patients are put on a machine that creates a vacuum to help drain the mucus and fluid that accumulates in a collapsed lung. It's the nurses' duty to empty that container every so often. After a while it wouldn't be out of the ordinary to be cleaning out the drainage jar with one hand while you're eating a cheese sandwich with the other!

* * *

In the cardiac ward, the patients stare at the heart monitor screens, as if by effort of will they can keep the beeping signal regular and strong. They always feel awkward and vulnerable when it's time to go home, and I remove the electrode pasties. They have so little faith in the restorative abilities of the body, or the resiliency of the heart. But they do go home. I'm pleased with God's design of the body and man's inventions to compliment that design.

Still, there's a lot of gloom and fear in the cardiac section of the hospital. Not from the staff, because we see progress every day, but from the patients, as this is the Big One. The heart has problems, and you can go quickly. I've often thought that's the way I want to go. Quick heart attack, and Boom! You're gone. No lingering chronic disease for me.

Better yet, a cerebral aneurism. A little headache, and Poof! You're gone.

* * *

Heart attacks seem to hit people unexpectedly. Never mind the years on the spare-ribs, beer, and Twinkies diet. When it hits, it's a wakeup call, and this awakening, as much as the damage to the heart muscle, seems to generate the mood and sobriety so prevalent on the cardiac wing.

It was refreshing then to come to work one day and find a patient who was upbeat and smiling. My first duty after receiving the shift report is to check everyone's vital signs. That's when I noticed the broad smile and palpable cheer of Mr. Thomas. His charm was so hypnotic that I took a few moments to go back and talk with him.

"Well, you sure do seem happy today. What's your secret?"

"Truth is, something happened last night" he confided. "I got a new attitude."

"What happened?" I asked, now curious.

"You see, I had another heart attack last night, after you went home. They called the crash cart in on me, and everybody was working on me. Maybe you heard of this thing called an out-of-body?"

My wide eyes encouraged him to go on.

"While they was workin' on me I wasn't there. I was up by the ceiling. I could see all around. I was looking down on them making all a fuss over me. Meanwhile, it's like I can see through the walls, and there's this beautiful garden. It was the most gorgeous place I ever seen. I'm walking along this path, and there's flowers and smells and music."

I did hear about out-of-body experiences. That was in the Death and Dying module in school. It's sometimes part of the near-death experience.

"I keep walking along this trail in the garden. The flowers are getting more beautiful, and the music is just wonderful the more I walk along. Then I come to an iron gate. I can see the garden past the iron gate, and it's even more beautiful, and I want to go there. At the same time I can look down and see them getting the paddles ready to shock my heart."

"I'm grabbing at the rails on this iron fence, trying to figure out how to get through there. The gate is not really iron. It's kind of gold colored and you can see part-way through it. Then there's two "Bangs." The first bang is me realizing these are the Pearly Gates. The second bang is the heart machine, and I'm zapped back into my body."

"Oh, my God! That's incredible! How do you feel now?"

"You know, it was real. It was the most real thing I ever seen. I don't care if I die, or if I have to stay here, 'cause I know where I'm going. I could go any time. That place was fantastic. But if I have to stay here a while longer, that's OK too."

* * *

They say psychics can see auras around people. Lights and energy swirl around their head and body. I've never seen an aura, but somehow things seemed brighter in that fellow's room. More than his words, his peace, his sense of joy spoke to me.

The next day I went out and bought a book I had heard of: ***Life After Life*** by Dr. Raymond Moody. I read that book several times. It was the Holy Grail I had been searching for. Between Mr. Thomas and Dr. Moody, the study of near-death experiences pretty much changed my life.

I'm not a religious person. I cannot go to one church every Sunday. But I love spiritual insight and metaphysics. Every once in a while I get a wave of Christian fervor. Opportunities for Christian service abound in nursing.

There was a kind old man on my unit. I was helping him get dressed. He was telling me how he was once a football player. Now his body was shrunken and frail. He joked about how his legs were like sticks now.

His feet smelled, so I decided to wash them before getting his shoes and socks on. Didn't Jesus wash his disciples' feet? I remember some woman washed the feet of Jesus and dried them with her hair. Maybe I could be of service to this withered old man.

How did Jesus cope with getting old? Oh, that's right, he was crucified.

"After two days in the hospital I took a turn for the nurse."
- W. C. Fields

WORKING

The first thing that hits you when applying for a job in nursing is that the hospital runs every day, day and night, all year long. Entry level positions usually involve the night shift. I've worked night shift, generally 11:00 PM to 7:00 AM, and that is actually easier than swing shift. If you're on night shift, you can still go out with friends in the evening before work. And the days I have off, I stay up late into the night, so the sleep schedule isn't too far off.

If you work swing shift you never have any social life. Everyone who works a regular day job is out of synch with you. Besides, you generally have to work at least one day of the weekend.

* * *

Nursing is serious work. You are literally responsible for someone's life. The entire shift was upset one evening when a beloved patient died. We all decided to go out for a drink in honor of Mr. D.

It's about midnight, and we all march into a local watering hole, still in our scrubs and white nursing uniforms. Everyone is a wee bit depressed over losing this really sweet old fellow. We raised a toast to him. Meanwhile, the nurses' uniforms triggered that universal fantasy in men, and the bar patrons started drifting over to our table, trying to pick up or dance with the girls. All of the girls, however, were in no mood to party. Finally, with one drunk and persistent player pestering her, a co-worker stood up, came over to me – the only male in the group – and loudly announced "Oh, our man won't let us dance with anyone else but him!"

That kept them at bay. The drunks thought it a real harem. The sober folks got the joke and got the message.

* * *

Hospitals offer acute care. You go to the hospital for a broken leg or a heart attack. Much of nursing however is for less than critical care. For institutions like Kaiser, a good portion of the medical care is provided at clinics. The third big medical sector is long-term care, such as nursing homes and assisted living facilities. Those nurses who get tired of the intensity of the acute care hospital will sometimes drift over to the clinics or nursing homes.

Hospitals have an emergency response called Code Blue. It means someone is not breathing and his complexion is turning blue. There are other codes in the hospital, such as Code Red for a fire. Nursing homes generally don't have the staff or machinery to respond to a heart attack or acute emergency. Instead the staff simply calls 911, and paramedics take the patient to the hospital. The biggest challenge for nursing home staff is deciding when to call in the paramedics. Certainly choking, a heart attack or stroke warrants such a call. Staffing at nursing homes isn't quite the same as at a hospital, so there are times when it's not clear if a condition is an emergency or not. A blood sugar crisis, for example can go either way.

One of my fellow nurses was a wee bit overwhelmed. She called 911 for a resident who was impacted: chronically constipated to the point where he was in pain. We made up a new moniker for that one: Code Brown.

* * *

Acute care nursing has all the glory, but the real angels of medicine are people who work in nursing homes. These nurses and assistants are the folks who will be taking care of your parents in the last years of their lives. They man the front lines in care for the elderly. With chronic understaffing and a focus on corporate profits, these dedicated people often work in deplorable conditions.

How sad, that the so-called golden years have become a nightmare for so many Americans. How cruel, that we treat our seniors so miserably, because some political strategist labels the services as "socialism."

* * *

Back in nursing school we had a module on nutrition, and how important food is in maintaining health.

At the end of one lecture the dietitian casually added, "Of course, the staff would never eat the patient's food!"

I remember thinking *Of course not!*

Zoom ahead 5 years. I'm working on the night shift at a major hospital. Most of the work is done in the first few hours. We settle in to do paperwork and midnight vital signs. During the day there's all kinds of activity. The teaching hospital has "rounds" for different medical specialties. The interns studying the kidneys for example might have Renal Rounds, visiting patients with kidney conditions. Then there's Cardiac Rounds, and Neurology Rounds.

Most of the hospital food, in fact pretty much everything except the entrée, is packaged in individual modules. There'd be a sealed cup of pudding for desert, a frozen individual serving of pizza, and small containers of juices, and deserts. I made up my own process called Refrigerator Rounds. Let's see, the fellow in room 211-B went into a coma earlier today. I guess he won't be needing that chocolate pudding.

* * *

You have a lot of opportunity as a nurse to go into related fields of medicine. One of my most enjoyable jobs was working as a telephone advice nurse to diabetic and cardiac patients. You have an opportunity to help people make informed decisions about their own health care. You can teach them about diet, exercise, and medications, and how they all work together.

The program I worked with provided regular calls to motivated people. They were often eager to get their next lessons. Even though it was telephone work, we got to know the participants, because they would enroll in a months-long program to learn about caring for their illness.

People are friendly for the most part, and it's fun talking with them. One particularly jovial fellow was telling me that he just celebrated his 50th wedding anniversary.

"Did you do anything special, Joe? I mean to mark your anniversary."

"Well, actually yes," he said. "I dressed up like Justin Timberlake and my wife had a wardrobe accident!"

* * *

You get all kinds of odd questions when you're a telephone advice nurse. One fellow asked how many calories you burn from having sex. We finally found an answer somewhere: about 250 calories. Naturally the subject generated a lot of humor and teasing among the staff nurses.

Joking with the nurse in the next cubicle I asked, "Does that mean that if I'm with four women at once that I'd burn up 1000 calories?"

"Yes, but if you're by yourself it's only 75 calories."

"Dang!"

"Love one another and help others to rise to the higher levels, simply by pouring out love. Love is infectious and the greatest healing energy."
- Sai Baba

TYPICAL DAY: Med/Surg

The medical/surgical unit is the mainstay of most hospitals. This is where people come when they have a serious illness, such as cancer, kidney failure, or physical trauma, such as a car accident. A wide variety of surgeries are performed on the Med/Surg unit. Some hospitals have separate wings for specialized surgery, such as cardiac surgery or orthopedics, but for the most part operations and invasive medical procedures are centered on the Med/Surg unit. This is where most acute care nursing takes place, and as a new nurse you can expect to spend time here.

I'm working the evening shift. I like this best. You don't get all the commotion and confusion of the day shift, with its two meals interrupting things, doctors' rounds demanding attention, and the 9-to-5 workers with all their "special" requirements. On the day shift you get more social workers, psychological counselors, specialist doctors making consultations, and procedures, such as EKGs, blood work, and Physical Therapy.

Surgery patients are generally admitted the day before their operation then they spend a few days recuperating before going home. The typical stay might be 3 or 4 days with the first day being preparations and examinations. The second day is the actual operation, often followed by a few hours in the Intensive Care Unit (ICU) or the Recovery Room. Finally they will need post-op bandage changes and monitoring.

Serious medical conditions often follow the same basic pattern; admission, exams and blood tests, X-rays, doctor visits, treatments, monitoring, and follow-up.

This repeating sequence of events for patients sets the tone for the start of the nurse's day. You start with the inter-shift report. The nurse assigned to the previous shift will describe the condition of the patients you will be working with.

You're generally assigned 6 to 8 patients, and the first thing you look for is where they are in the admission-to-discharge cycle. Two empty beds means you'll probably be getting at least one admission. The admission exam takes a lot of time, but it's generally easy work, with an emphasis on making the patient comfortable and getting him oriented to procedures and operations of the staff. You have to read up on his history, the expected procedures, and the nursing care plan. There is usually a family member to work with too.

The day-of-operation patients require the most attention. You have to have the pre-op medications squared away in a timely manner. These are large, powerful injections, and you have to build in enough flexibility to accommodate the sometimes shifting schedule of the surgeons. Likewise, when they first come out of surgery, or the recovery room, they need focused attention. The doctor writes post-op orders, and there's usually a curve-ball or two which requires quick thinking and extra work for the nurse. Example: during the operation the patient developed a short-term cardiac arrhythmia, and the doctor wants to schedule an electrocardiogram and a consult with a cardiologist. This is accomplished through some phone calls and paper-work, but it also entails revisions to the nurses' notes, the patient care plan, and interaction with family members.

The last few days of an admission are the easiest. The procedures and the work load are not as intense. The patient is a lot calmer and is looking forward to going home. His medical status is generally improving, and he's getting more visitors. He's now rid of the anxiety so common before surgery. His IV gets taken out. His doctor is making follow-up visits, and that scar on his abdomen is healing well.

So, now I get the report. I have 4 rooms to cover and 7 patients. One room has two empty beds with one admission expected. The new admission is just arriving as report begins, but the Nursing Assistants are handling the preparations while the nurses give the shift report. This means I will have to talk to the admission patient right away, even before I collect vital signs on the others. I have just one day-of-operation patient, and he's gotten back at 1:00 PM. It's 4:00 PM now, and he's stable, alert, with no emergencies pending. The other 5 patients are all stable post-op. They are the same ones I've worked with yesterday, so it looks like a good, easy shift. I get the report on their blood work values, what the doctors have changed on their medications, and which procedures are required. For 3 out of the 5 post-op patients I have bandage changes, which is a sterile procedure, and I usually ask for help with from a Nursing Assistant or fellow nurse.

In this particular facility, the division of labor is such that a senior registered nurse, an RN, handles the IVs, the pre-op medications, and the patient care plans, while less experienced nurses are assigned to patient rooms. In California, the two-year nursing program gets you a Licensed Vocational Nurse degree, which is the same as a Licensed Practical Nurse in other states. RN degrees on the other hand require 4 or 5 years of college.

I make a note to myself to ask one of the Nursing Assistants to help me with the dressing changes. It's great to have good rapport with them, and we often exchange favors to make life easier on the unit. I help them with bed linen changes, getting patients to the bathroom, and with meals. They assist me with paper work, vital signs, and certain medical procedures, like changing out a Foley (urine collection) bag.

Many NAs are planning to become nurses themselves, or else they are nurses in their heart or motivations, but don't have the diploma to make it official. I love them. They get the lowest pay, spend the most hands-on time with patients, get all the ass-wipe jobs (literally), and yet remain on the low end of the prestige hierarchy. Except, that is, for the housekeeping staff; yet another wonderful group of unsung heroes.

Immediately after the shift report conference, I go to the room where the new patient is arriving. The Nursing Assistants have put away his clothes and gotten him into his hospital gown. I have gathered all the paper-work for his admission, stopping off to read the doctors' orders, his medical history, and his medications. I introduce myself to him and his wife. There is an exchange of pleasantries, and a social worker arrives. The social worker needs to talk to them about financial matters. She requests 15 minutes alone with them. I agree. This gives me time to collect vital signs on the other patients.

I make my way to the other rooms, collecting blood pressure readings, pulse, respirations, and a general visual evaluation of each patient. This is a good time. I know most of them from previous days, and as I take their vital signs I check on their mood, what's happened to them in the last day or so, and make them feel comfortable. The vital signs procedure lets me feel their skin, look into their eyes, and check for cardiac arrhythmias. I scan their bandages too. Sometimes if there is an excess discharge, I'll need to change the bandage more often than is posted in the nursing notes.

The 15 minutes are up, and I make my way back to the new admission. There are forms to fill out and a bunch of questions for both him and his wife. The monotony and the volume of the questions on the admission forms actually help him to calm down and get comfortable with me. During this time I do a general body exam too. I look for past scars, rashes, or anything unusual. His skin seems a bid red and flushed to me, especially on his face and chest. Then I smell alcohol on his breath. He may have been drinking prior to admission.

For many admissions we have to give a TB test; a small, subcutaneous injection. I go to the nurses' station to prepare the injection, and I check his chart again while there. Then I see it in his history; "ETOH," which is medical short-hand for alcohol abuse. Somehow I missed that among the alphabet soup of medical abbreviations in his history. I will have to be more careful and thorough when I read a patients' history.

Back at his room, his wife is standing outside, and I take the opportunity to ask about his drinking. She admits that he "had a few" prior to coming to the hospital. I make a note to myself to be sure to include this in my nursing notes and in the report to the next shift. His drinking means he may be very nervous about the hospital stay, and that he may be going through withdrawal while here, not to mention the many medical problems associated with alcoholism.

Vital signs are finished and I record them in patient charts, to get a head-start on nursing notes at the end of shift. I've made a couple passes to the rooms to chat with everyone and get started on medications.

Medications are a major part of nursing. It's so crucial that you quickly learn the names of the major drugs, their functions, their side effects, dosages, generic names, and interactions. Every once in a while a doctor throws in a new one, and you have to go check the books to get up to speed. Depending on the type of nursing you're involved with, you'll see a remarkably consistent spectrum of meds; anti-anxiety drugs, pain-killers, drugs for high blood pressure and high cholesterol. In the surgery unit stool softeners are common, not just for constipation, but abdominal surgery prevents the patient from bearing down for bowel movements, and the stool softener mitigates that problem.

Many of the meds are easier to take with food, so much of what is scheduled for 4:00 PM, 5:00 PM or 6:00 PM are given with the evening meal. Diabetic tests, blood sugar levels, though must be checked before meals, as eating affects blood glucose levels.

The Nursing Assistants do most of the work at meal times. After dinner I change the bandages and make notes on anything unusual. Everything looks good. Three of the bandage changes are done, and the wounds are healing well. I talk to the patients as I change their dressings. Most are surprised how resilient the body is. Things heal quickly. They get better and go home. It's an uplifting process.

The last bandage change is the most difficult. This is the one I ask the nursing assistant for help with. I gather all the supplies and lay out the sterile field. The patient's wound is deeper than normal, and is healing more slowly than expected. It is progressing, however, and there are no signs of infection. I have to soak gauze pads in a solution that is half strength hydrogen peroxide. With sterile gloves, I dip the gauze in the peroxide solution and pack it inside the wound, then cover it with a thick dry dressing.

As I'm packing up and cleaning the area, a nurse-supervisor comes in and gives the patient a requested pain pill. The other nurse picks up the paper cup with the peroxide solution in it, thinking it's water, and gives it to him to wash down the pill.

Before I can stop him, he's swallowed the pill and a few gulps of peroxide.

Whoops! This is a major incident. We have to write up an incident report. In such a situation there's a great deal of embarrassment and finger-pointing. The real concern, as we learned in nursing school, is not the egos of the staff involved, but rather patient safety. Was he in any danger from swallowing a half-strength peroxide solution? We look it up in the books and consult the doctor. It turns out not be a serious error. In fact half-strength peroxide solution is used as an oral rinse for treating gum and tongue sores. Swallowing a little is not too dangerous. The doctor orders that we observe the patient for any side effects over the next 24 hours, but nothing happens and the patient is discharged two days later.

Still, I get written up for a nursing error. I should have used a bowl instead of a paper cup for the peroxide solution. This weighs on me. Errors, especially medication errors can get you fired, and it can affect your entire career as well as your nursing license. I vow to myself to be more careful in the future. I'm pissed though. The supervising nurse was involved too. I got written up but she didn't. No one said life is fair.

We're approaching late night now. The patients are put to bed between 9:00 and 10:00 PM, so that gives me time to finish charting. I have to include the peroxide incident, the new patient with alcohol on his breath, and of course all the vital signs and bandage changes.

There were no major emergencies on this shift. I worked well with all the patients and the other staff. Soon it's time for the night shift to check in. I give my report, confessing now to the peroxide incident and the new patient with alcohol on his breath. All-in-all it was a good evening. Nobody died and I didn't get fired.

> *"Eventually you will come to understand that love heals everything, and love is all there is."*
> - Gary Zukav

TYPICAL DAY: Clinic

Acute care hospitals are where all the action is. You are immersed in emergencies, and you can move up the ranks quickly by acquiring new skills and through exposure to state of the art technology. Some nurses, however are attracted to clinical nursing because it offers regular workdays, 8 to 5 PM or thereabouts, and you usually have weekends free. Often too, the doctors have bankers' hours, and may be around only from 9 to 4 PM, so the real work period is short, regular, and relatively low anxiety, compared to acute care.

There are all kinds of clinics and much of medical care is now provided through these specialized facilities. Many are located in a medical business park right next to the acute care hospital, so there can be a gradual, seamless transition from a medical emergency to more long term care.

Clinics specialize in cancer treatments, back care, ophthalmology, orthopedics, dermatology, OB/Gyn, diabetes treatment, physical therapy, psychological counseling, weight loss and nutrition, and a whole spectrum of specialized medical services. There are, in addition, many medical facilities that are similar to clinics but serve different segments of the population. These include exam and drug screening centers for business new-hires, urgent care centers, dialysis facilities, drug and alcohol treatment programs, and podiatry, to name a few.

In addition to having a regular day-time schedule, nurses are sometimes drawn to these clinics and facilities because they offer specialized career training. Some nurses, for example, might work with diabetes patients, which requires specific knowledge and treatments, and then it's logical for them to ease over to a diabetes treatment center. The clinics also foster working with a select group of doctors and nurses, or focusing on a particular science. Others nurses, for spiritual reasons, might choose to work at a hospice dedicated to treating those with a terminal illness.

I've worked in a few clinic-style settings.
One was at a hemodialysis center. It didn't
last long.

Hemodialysis is a very specialized function,
and I was required to take an intensive class
on kidney function, diet, and the operation
of the dialysis machine. I found this
fascinating but a little scary at the same
time.

Poorly controlled diabetes and other
diseases can cause kidney failure. Severe
cases result in what they call End Stage
Renal Disease, or ESRD. When the kidneys
don't work properly, all kinds of toxins build
up in the blood. A very strict diet can help
prevent the buildup of these toxins, but no
matter how self-disciplined a patient is, he
still needs to have dialysis treatments two or
three times a week.

In the most common form of dialysis, two
large bore needles are placed in the patient,
one to withdraw blood and the other to
return it. The blood circulates through the
dialysis machine where is it cleaned by a
process of osmosis. Blood chemistry and the
patient's vital signs are monitored
constantly. The science of the process is

awe-inspiring, but the chronic, dependent nature of the sessions can be depressing, both for the nurse and the patient. The only real alternative, besides dying, is to get a kidney transplant. Once they get a transplant, the improvement is both instant and remarkable.

I left after just a few weeks not because of the work, but because of the schedule. Most clinic shifts are 8 or 9 hours long. A recent trend though is to move to 12-hour shifts. The employers like this because they can extend the hours of the clinic, and the employees like it because they can work just 3 days a week, 36 hours, and get paid the equivalent of a 40-hour work week. These are long, difficult days, but then you have plenty of off-time too.

Unbelievably, some nurses hold down two separate jobs of 3-day, 12-hour shifts. This may be possible for some dynamic young whipper-snappers, but I entered the nursing profession as a result of a mid-life crisis, and just one shift of 12 hours was out there at the extremes of my physical abilities.

The clinic will cram as many patients as they can into the day, so you're monitoring several patients simultaneously. This is intense. Some days we have to prepare a huge vat of cleaning solution that is run through the dialysis machines between treatments. The preparation of the cleaning solution takes a few hours in the morning and requires precise measurements and testing for pH levels. You do feel more like a swimming pool cleaning technician at this point, and suddenly the 12-hour shift is more like 14 hours.

The dialysis machines are complicated, with lots of tubes and dials and buttons. If you make a mistake and push the wrong button, you could easily end the life of the patient. It's not likely, but it IS possible to push the cleaning solution into the veins of the patient killing him instantly. There were a few times where I pressed the wrong buttons or adjusted the dials to the wrong setting, but I always caught the error in time.

With the long shifts, the extra hours to mix the cleaning batch, and the high intensity levels of the treatments, I calculated that it was only a matter of time before I made a mistake that would truly endanger a patient. I decided this was not the line of work for me. I did find work at another facility that had the regular 8-hour shifts. It wasn't in the hemodialysis arena, but the knowledge I gained from the dialysis center about kidney function helped me in my career from then on.

* * *

A more successful episode in my career was the Orthopedics Clinic. Once I knew I wanted to explore working in the clinics, I resigned as a full-time Med/Surg nurse and took a job as "On-call" nurse at the clinic. This work is less steady, but it was all day-time shifts, and allowed me to work at the clinics on an as-needed basis. I liked the Ortho clinic because the patients were not really sick, but rather suffered some kind of trauma or broken bone. After a few shifts there, I switched over to full-time Ortho Clinic nurse. Again I was given a short but intensive on-the-job training course where I learned to apply plaster casts to broken limbs, take them off, fit people for crutches, and assist doctors with procedures.

A typical day at the Ortho clinic is low stress, even fun at times. The people with broken bones are generally younger than Med/Surg patients, and there is not a lot of blood, gore, or pain involved, not at the treatment stage, anyway.

I'd be at the clinic at 8:00 AM, and go immediately to the day's assignment schedule. There were 5 or 6 orthopedic doctors and surgeons there with a full schedule of patients visiting for follow-up care, mostly to have casts removed. There were others who had surgery that day and would need a cast put on. There were also

unscheduled jobs from the Emergency
Room. After a few days I got to know all the
doctors. The clinics can be fun because you
are working closely with doctors, and there
is the occasional slow day where you get to
relax for a while.

This Ortho Clinic was merged with a
Podiatry Clinic in the same facility. I start
off by checking the charts of the scheduled
patients. In the morning I have 3 cast
removals, one on an elbow, one forearm,
and one foot. In the afternoon I assist a
doctor with a compound fracture treatment
of someone's leg.

By the time I finish reading the charts the
first patients are arriving. The elbow cast is
on a young boy who fell off a skate board.
Kids are terrified of the cast-removal saw. I
show the boy how it works. It's a circular
saw something like a Dremel tool, but the
blade doesn't spin; it jiggles back and forth
just a fraction of an inch. So if it touches
your skin, the skin just moves like Jello. If it
touches the solid cast, it blasts it to
smithereens. I show him by touching my
own hand to the blade, then the edge of his
cast. They all say the same thing when the
cast comes off at the end of a few weeks:
"Whoa! That feels so weird!"

Before the next scheduled patient arrives,
we get a hairline ulna (forearm) fracture

71

from the Emergency Room. Sometimes the attending doctor applies the cast, but this time he's busy with other patients. He knows me, and leaves me to do the cast alone, having seen I don't need supervision. I go get a pail of warm water and the supplies. I clean the boys' skin and wrap it with a soft, felt-like roll. I then dip the plaster rolls, one by one, in the warm water and wrap them around his wrist, up between his thumb and fingers and down to near the elbow. I smooth out all the sharp edges and add a little extra to the bottom where I know he'll be resting it on the desk at school. The doctor pops back in to check my work.

The other cast removals are on adults, and they are not as impressed with the oscillating saw as the kids are. They are glad to be rid of the weeks-long burden of the weight of the plaster, and again I get the "Wow, that feels so strange!" comments.

It's lunch time. I usually eat in the hospital cafeteria. The food is good and at a decent price. I work with another male nurse, and we've taken to wearing the ubiquitous dull blue scrubs that the surgeons wear. The application and removal of casts gets dust and debris all over our uniforms, so the scrubs work well at savings on uniform costs. Wearing the blue scrub outfits we are almost always viewed as doctors by visitors to the cafeteria. We're often engaged in conversation by these visitors, and we chuckle to ourselves in the deception, wallowing in the adoration.

After lunch I greet patient at the curb and get him into a wheelchair. He's had a compound fracture of the lower leg, breaking both the tibia and fibula. I wheel him into the doctors' office. His lower leg is encircled by steel rings, with rods going right into his flesh at regular intervals. "Skewered" is the only way to describe it. I help the doctor clean off the minute scabs where the rods enter his skin. The scars from the fracture and the surgery are bulbous and pink two weeks after the accident. Everything is healing well, and I'm surprised when the patient mentions that he is almost completely free of pain. The X-rays reveal just as much hardware inside his leg as outside, and you can see what looks like common wood screws holding his bones in place. As I wheel him back out to the car we discuss how amazing the body is at healing.

The afternoon is slow and the supervisor switches my assignment from the casts and crutches to the Podiatry side of the clinic. Podiatry is not as interesting medically, as it consists mostly of women torturing their own feet by forcing them into too-small shoes that twist their bones at odd angles.

The main tasks here are setting up sterile fields for the doctors, cleaning the feet of the patients, and cleaning up the mess afterwards. Most of the procedures are corn removals and nail and skin care. This would normally be a dull assignment, but in this clinic the two podiatrists are real comedians, and they seem to be engaged in a contest as to who can make their patients laugh the hardest.

The rest of the day is filled with simple procedures, off-color jokes, and patients flirting with their doctors. It's a very pleasant day. *Ha! I get paid for this?*

"Drugs are not always necessary. Belief in recovery always is."
- Norman Cousins

TYPICAL DAY: Nursing Home

Nursing homes get a bad rap. It's true that some of them are merely warehouses for the elderly, and a mark of shame for the nation, as we treat our senior citizens with such disrespect. Many facilities are run strictly for business purposes, so that funding and staffing is at a minimum, while profits are worshiped by corporate shareholders. Counterbalancing this trend is the professionalism of the staff, their dedication, and their heart-felt motivation to providing quality care.

Most families who have to put an elderly parent into a home know of the hard choices involved. Fortunately there is a growing wave of awareness of this situation as the US population ages, and many nursing homes are answering the challenge with well designed facilities and a commitment to the quality of life of their residents.

From the nurses' perspective, you know you can always find work pretty much anywhere in the country, and you can choose to work anywhere from one day a week to full-time.

The staffing structure at a nursing home is totally different from both hospital work and the clinical setting. Doctors are not around much. They make scheduled visits and consults to see their patients in the nursing home, and much of the time the licensed nurses have to call the doctor's office for questions and medication changes. Nurses are focused primarily on medications and injections in the nursing home setting. Most of the patient care is handled by the Nursing Assistants.

As a nurse my main task is to get the medications to all the patients. In a nursing home you might be assigned anywhere from 25 to 40 patients on a wing. You are aided by a group of Nursing Assistants who do the hands-on work.

I've chosen to work the evening shift three days a week. I like evenings because you have to deal with just one meal, and the patients are in bed for a few hours at the end of the shift, so you have time to do charting.

The shift starts, as usual, with the nursing report from the day workers. There's not a lot of turnover in nursing homes. Sometimes there's an admission, or a resident goes out to the hospital for some emergency or procedure. Today I have a patient who has gone out to a dialysis center for a treatment, and she should be back soon.

There are two empty rooms, and I hope there are no admissions. A new admission takes up a lot of time, and it usually comes during those busy hours between 4:00 and 6:00 PM.

The report indicates everyone is stable. A few have requested pain pills during the day, and a few need bandages changed, but for the most part it's dispensing meds that takes up my time.

When report is over I count the narcotics with the nurse from the previous shift. I make quick rounds to say hello to everyone and give the Nursing Assistants their assignments. Generally, they regulate themselves and have preferences for which rooms they want to cover. I try to give them some freedoms to choose patients and rooms, as everyone has their favorites. There's a new male orderly assigned to me, and he takes some extra attention.

Next it's the med cart. Nursing home work centers around the med cart, which I push from room to room. The immediate concern is the 4:00 PM meds, and I get these into little cups as quickly as possible, running from cart to patient to deliver them. Most of the patients know the routine, so it's simple. The cart is organized with drawers and spaces for each patient. Medications for each patient are on cards in their individual slots. Some meds though have their own "special" place, which was a real pain to learn when I first started. The bulk drugs like Tylenol are kept in a common area in the top drawer. Then ear drops, eye drops, lotions, and topical ointments may be in another "special" place, not to mention those in the refrigerator.

Drawing the meds from their containers, checking the dosages and labels, putting them in cups, and delivering them to the right people is the bulk of the work. There is a round of meds for 4:00 PM, 6:00 MP, 8:00 PM and occasionally at off-hour times. Each patient requires finding the right drawer and slot, doing deep knee bends as you locate them, and locking up the cart when you leave it.

Some patients have mental or physical conditions which interfere with taking medications, and these have to be given during the evening meal, sometimes mixed with their food. The first few weeks on the job you learn who these patients are, and their meds are held for mealtime.

The next big race is the pre-meal blood sugar tests for diabetic patients. The amount of their medications depends on their blood sugar levels just prior to eating, so I have to rush and do a bunch of finger sticks, blood tests, and drawing up of the correct amount of insulin for them. This is a very intensive, time-consuming, and critical process. Some have to be tested again after dinner, or before bedtime. Some diabetics are "brittle," meaning their sugar levels can fluctuate wildly depending on what they eat and their level of activity. These take the most attention.

Meanwhile, the NAs are getting everyone to the dining room for dinner. There are always a few people who want to eat in their room or who need help with cutting the food and eating, so everyone is busy until about 6:30 when they settle back into the rooms. There are some evening activities in common areas that the alert residents participate in. Others just go from their bed to a wheelchair, to dinner, and back to bed.

Every once in a while someone falls out of a chair or gets a cut. Their skin is thin and tears easily. Each such incident requires immediate attention, and I have to fill out an incident report. The skin tears need to be bandaged and documented. All the while I continue to push the cart around to each room, following up on the nightly meds and last-minute blood sugar tests.

All during the shift the NAs come to me with questions, little emergencies, and personnel problems. They relay the requests for pain pills and sleeping pills.

Narcotics and certain pills are locked in a cabinet at the nursing station, so each pain-pill request is a trip down the hall, some paper work, and a personal visit to the patient.

Most people are back in bed by 9:00 PM and I take this time to catch up on patient assessments, phone calls to family members, and rounds where I perform skin treatments, bandage changes, and general interaction with the residents. By 10:00 PM I can start charting and making notes for the next shift.

Some residents have to be up early for doctor appointments, outside treatments, or family events, so I want to prepare notes for the inter-shift report.

It was a good day. There were no major emergencies, and no admissions to upset the schedule.

I have to record all the incidents, the skin tears, the doctor requests, and the special appointments for the next day. As the shift report approaches, I gather the NAs and ask if there is anything I need to know. It's a good crew.

As I mentioned elsewhere, the NAs are the great unsung heroes of medical care, especially in nursing homes. They do all the grunt work, get low pay, and little recognition. I know, somewhere deep inside, there is a God who appreciates this, and that his words are true: The first shall be last, and the last shall be first.

"Bad administrative arrangements often make it impossible to nurse."
- Florence Nightingale

DOWNERS

On every shift I take vital signs of the patients at least once. On the cardiac ward it's important to actually feel the pulse and listen to the heart sounds. The stethoscope on the chest reveals important details. You can hear breath sounds. Often with continued bed rest, the lungs can fill up and cause gurgling, rales, or other breathing noises. You hear the heartbeat, and you can begin to tell from the rhythm and strength how the heart is doing. An irregular heartbeat is cause for concern. The most common problem is atrial fibrillation. This is a condition where the upper chambers, the atria, beat at a different rate than the ventricles, the bigger chambers. Sometimes the atria beat at exactly twice the rate of the ventricles. The radial pulse then might be

60 beats per minute, but the stethoscope on the chest will register 120 beats. Less commonly, you might hear a very irregular atrial rhythm with a more-or-less steady ventricular beat.

The hospital I started with was a teaching hospital. Interns passed through the halls every day. Some of the nurses have been on the unit for years; many more years than the interns. Quite regularly then, we'd have nurses watching the heart monitors at the nursing station who knew a lot more about EKG readings than the doctors on duty. Just looking at the video screen of the heart rhythm you begin to learn what to look for: the regularity of the beats; the spacing between the atrial contraction and the ventricular, what they call the P-Q interval.

Some of the lazier nurses would just look at the heart monitor to record vital signs. Those monitors cannot always be trusted however. I once had a patient with three different pulse rates. Feeling his radial pulse I counted 66 beats. Listening to his chest I heard 132 beats. He had atrial fib at exactly twice the ventricular rate. Looking at the monitor his pulse showed 80 beats with no atrial fib. The man's electrodes had come undone, and somehow his heart monitor was picking up the signal from the patient in the next bed. The lesson is, you have to make a hands-on examination.

* * *

I had a psychiatric patient once. He had
both medical and mental problems. In
reading his chart, I noticed (the first time
for me) that he had an order for a placebo
shot if he complained of pain. A placebo
shot is simple saline solution that has no
active medicinal ingredients. The patient
simply thinks he is getting a powerful
narcotic. To me his pain seemed real, with
sweating and irritable behavior. I gave him
the shot and he was immediately relieved.

This process, giving a placebo, can cause a
disconnect in any thinking person. Is the
mind really capable of generating pain? Is it
also capable of relieving that pain? Big
questions. Whole new ballgame.

I had another patient, a heart surgery case.
He was Hawaiian. He was not doing too
well. One day about 20 members of his
family arrived from across the sea and
performed a faith healing. After the
ceremony, they sang a Hawaiian song;
something I hadn't heard before or since.
Maybe it was a genuine native creation,
because you could hear waves of music,
growing, swelling, subsiding, and
overlapping just like ocean waters. The next
day he popped out of bed and started
making preparations to go home. He fully

recovered. I think the music made a big difference.

* * *

New patients get a lot of attention. Their stress level goes down considerably if you take a few extra moments to stay with them, answer their questions, and get them oriented to the unit.

One fellow was new on my shift, and I held a long conversation with him, as I filled out the some admission forms. I took his vital signs, which were normal. Then I noticed he was admitted with the primary diagnosis of high blood pressure. That was pretty rare. Usually doctors treat their people as outpatients for high blood pressure. The cardiac unit was reserved for more severe problems, like valve disease or arrhythmias. His blood pressure was 136/86; not that bad. I thought I'd better check it again.

As I got the cuff on his arm, the man's wife walked into the room.

"Well, did you get to talk to the doctor yet?" she bellowed at her husband.

"No, I just got here about an . . ."

"We have to know what he plans to do while you're here," she interrupted.

His blood pressure shot up to an alarming 212/118; right up there in stroke-out territory.

Later on that day, I ran across the man's doctor.

"Isn't it obvious," I asked, "that his blood pressure problems have their root in his confrontational relationship with his wife?"

"Yes, that's true," the doctor replied.

"Why then isn't he being treated with some kind of marriage counseling or psychotherapy?"

"Yes, that is a long-term approach. You have to realize this relationship with his spouse has been developing for over 30 years. We can't undo that in a short hospital stay. For the time being, we just have to give him medications that will treat the acute condition and hope he doesn't pop a blood vessel before the long-term treatment starts to show some effect."

"Well, hasn't medicine missed the boat if all we can do in the hospital is a quick fix?"

As soon as the words came out I realized that it was a rather harsh indictment of the medical profession. At the same time the doctor could see my point.

We both raised our eyebrows and presented a twisted smile towards each other. It was some kind of non-verbal agreement to call a truce on this matter.

Still, the pharmaceutical approach to a chronic social disorder troubled me. I began to wonder, even with all our knowledge of physiology, if the haggard husband might not be better served by forcing him to face up to the nagging by his wife.

"What would you have us do?" the doctor had asked me. "Withhold medicine that might save his life?"

Mmm! I don't know. What kind of life is being saved?

* * *

The anorexia patient isn't improving very well. One of the nurses has befriended her and confided in her. That's a good sign. The nurse tells the staff that the anorexia patient likes to eat, like at a party. They decide to organize a party in the staff lounge. The kitchen staff, though helpful, only has access to lame, institutional level pizzas, so we all chip in and order a real pizza, real soda and chips. Everyone is having a good time, but stealing secret glances to see if the anorexic girl eats anything. We all have good cheer and an upbeat attitude, but the girl only takes a few sips of soda.

The next day, I'm taking her vital signs. She is just lying there, naked. I'm losing it. I'm mad at her.

"What's wrong with you? Those girls spent a lot of time and expense on your party, and you don't even have the decency to take one bite?!"

No response. Vital signs are done now, but I persist.

"Didn't you have a good time? Did you even say 'Thank You' for the presents?"

No response; not even eye contact.

"What the fuck is wrong with you? You're just a spoiled little bastard!" And with that I stormed out.

I felt terrible later. I had never cursed a patient before. Anorexia disorders often go hand in hand with low self esteem. I probably set her back 10 years with that outburst. Still, it felt good to express the frustration. Sometimes I think a person needs a good kick in the butt instead of medical care. The guilt stayed with me for a while. With it came the first questions about the good I was doing, or not doing, as a nurse. It was the first drops of doubt.

* * *

Another time a patient came from a hovel. The clean sheets and the kind attention was an experience this woman had not known for many years. I came into her room to inform her that the doctor had just signed the orders. She could go home the next morning.

"Oh, no!" she blurted out.

"Don't you want to go home?"

"Well . . ."

Then I remembered reading her chart. She was admitted with a long list of vague but not life-threatening symptoms. Maybe this was one of those Münchausen syndrome cases. People are so starved for affection they make themselves sick, subconsciously or not, just to get medical attention. Another drop in the bucket of doubt.

Certainly I've had cases where the patient rings the bell every few minutes, just to have someone to talk to. The idea of making yourself sick, just for the strokes of human kindness; well, that's a bit much. What's the proper response to a situation like that? Isn't it a form of blackmail? And yet, like a medical condition, it's a call for help. What mean spirited SOB would *deny* someone that request? Should my response to the phony medical request include a lecture?

"Hi Mrs. Johnson. You rang the call bell? Is there something I can help you with?

"Yes, it's this IV. I think it's leaking. It doesn't feel right."

"Let me see. Mmm! There's no leaking, no swelling. It's just normal saline. There's no medications in the IV that would cause any pain. It's going in at the right rate. No, I think it's all OK."

"Oh, hi Mrs. Johnson. Fluff your pillow? Ok, here you go.

"Hello Mrs. Johnson. You called?

"Can you check this IV? I don't think it's running right."

Drip, drip, drip.

* * *

I was working in a nursing home. About half the residents were lucid and well functioning. The other half were either out

91

of it mentally, or confined to bed. Every once in a while the facility would host some kind of themed event, like "Moonlight Serenade" featuring a catered dinner and musical entertainment. But this dinner would be above and beyond the cost of living in the home. Consequently the families would be asked to sponsor the patient to the tune of $50 to $100 each. The patients really seemed to enjoy it.

During one such dinner I had a medication problem that required the signature of the head nurse. I couldn't find her. Finally someone told me that top supervisors were in the staff lounge. I entered the lounge to get her sign-off, and there in front of me were all the execs and supervisors, sitting down to a catered dinner, the exact same meal being served to the residents. So we had 22 servings for execs and 42 for the patients. Some deal.

These same executives and supervisors got a directive from corporate headquarters. A friend in the IT Department leaked the memo to the working staff. Every department head who comes in under budget for the year would get a $10,000 Christmas bonus. Every department head who comes in more than $50,000 under budget would receive a $25,000 Christmas bonus. There's only one way to save that much money: cut staffing.

* * *

The first wake-up call in a nursing career is that it's mostly shift work. If you have several years of experience and can move up the chain of command you might get a cushy day-shift position. Of course the real work of a nursing home is round the clock care. I worked the evening shift. Nursing home care is easier in the sense that there are far fewer emergencies and critical care issues. It's mostly tending to diabetic needs, cleanliness, and skin problems. The elderly have thin skin, and any little scratch can require attention and bandaging. On the down side, you have to take care of more than 30 patients at once, instead of the 6 or 8 you get in a hospital. Of course the Nursing Assistants do most of the grunt work, but the nurse has to get the medications out, and check blood sugars for the diabetic patients.

The biggest challenge on the evening shift is the 5:00 PM medications. Many patients are resistant to taking pills, and the evening meal provides an opportunity to mix the medications with food. Before dinner I have to draw several medications for each patient. I have to perform a finger stick on over half of them to check their blood sugar levels, and then prepare the right dosage of insulin for their shot. Some of the diabetic patients are what they call *brittle*. Their blood sugars soar up and down depending on what they eat, their level of activity, and God knows what else. Their care requires focused attention. Too much of a swing in blood sugar can result in a coma or death.

The two hours between 4:00 PM and 6:00 PM therefore are incredibly busy. It's unimaginable then that the day shift supervisors tend to schedule new admissions in the 5:00 PM time slot. That's exactly the hour they go home, and when I have the least time.

An admission demands several hours of personal attention. The admission, being the first impression of the facility, involves orienting the patient, answering questions and concerns of the family members, providing a medical entrance exam, and of course volumes of paperwork.

When they started scheduling admissions regularly at the 5:00 PM slot I complained. I wrote a detailed explanation of how that endangers the lives of diabetes patients. It happened again, so I wrote another letter, indicating I would leave if it occurred again. The next day I had TWO admissions, one at 5:00 PM and one at 6:00 PM. I quit.

I found out months later that the nurse who replaced me also quit for the same reason:

admissions during the dinner hour. Management finally heard. They hired a nurse whose sole function was to admit new patients. Sometimes you have to vote with your feet.

* * *

I applied for work at a nicer nursing home, one closer to my house. There's no nice way to say this, but a male nurse has a tremendous advantage in getting hired. So many residents believe you're a doctor, and so many procedures require strength, that there is a distinct advantage for a male nurse.

This job application consisted of three separate people interviewing me, followed by a brief review consisting of all three of them and myself. While I'm waiting for that final blessing, I felt on top of the world. Their smiling faces, nodding heads, and engaging discussions all pointed to me getting hired. As I waited I noticed a piano in the lobby, and as was my custom in the previous home, I sat down and belted out a few of the favorite Baptist hymns I had learned way back when. I knew from experience that the residents just love that good old-time religious music.

The staff calls me in for what I'm sure is the final formality of hiring.

95

"Oh, just one more question. Why did you leave your last job?"

I told them the full story of the 5:00 PM admissions, adding that adequate staffing is a top priority of mine. As my story unfolded, the approving nods seemed to disappear, and the smiles were replaced by open-mouthed shock. I guess I hit a nerve. Maybe this place didn't have adequate staffing either. Maybe they scheduled all their admission in the evenings.

I didn't get hired. Maybe I'll look into clinical work again. More voting with my feet.

"It's when we start working together that the real healing takes place... it's when we start spilling our sweat, and not our blood."
- David Hume

IS NURSING RIGHT FOR YOU?

Is nursing the right career choice for you? Only you can decide. I hope the previous chapters have provided an insight as to the nature of the work, the challenges, inspirations, and rewards you can get from nursing.

There are whole books and dedicated aptitude tests to help you decide if you're suited to this work. In the meantime, let me summarize what I see as the major variables in this occupation.

First and foremost, nursing offers steady work, decent pay, and job security. With Baby Boomers reaching retirement age there is a growing need for nurses. All the job surveys reveal that a medical career will guarantee you employment.

You can choose to work full-time, part-time, or on call. You have the opportunity to travel. You can work anywhere in the country, and even in foreign countries.

Second, the work can be fascinating. Whether you're interested in the workings of the human body, the potential for psychological healing, the science of pharmacology, electronics, microbiology, or research, you can easily find a rewarding niche within nursing to satisfy your inquisitive mind.

Third, nursing is a personally rewarding career. You help people when they need it most. You are up close and personal. There is nothing as intimate as working with a person wrestling with body image issues, with life and death decisions, and ultimately with the meaning of it all.

If you are spiritually or ethically inclined towards helping others, you will find great accomplishments in this field.

There are downsides too. With a business focus on profits, and the ever-present threat of financial down-turns, the staffing and support for patient care can suffer. You may find yourself questioning how people can suffer just so others can profit.

Along the same lines, the work can be depressing. You are often faced with pain and distress with few resources to cope with it. You need a strong foundation in your own faith, religion, or world-view in order to provide the physical, mental, and spiritual support that your patients so desperately seek.

On one level, you can be overwhelmed. From another perspective, you can look back and say you've done your best, and hope in some small way you've made a difference in someone's life.

"A merry heart doeth good like medicine."
- Proverbs 17:22

A NEW ERA

Nursing has changed a lot since I first went to school. In fact, the entire medical profession has changed. The new emphasis is on preventive health care and individual responsibility.

The old model was *I'm sick; you fix me.* The new model is *I'm sick, what have I been doing wrong? Maybe I'm not eating right or getting enough exercise.*

One of my most recent jobs was working as a telephone advice nurse, teaching people to care for their diabetic conditions. It's very rewarding to see people learn how to take control over their health. Maybe it's just one out of 100 patients, but when you hear a success story it makes the whole effort worthwhile.

One patient told me, "You know I feel so much better now. I don't have that blurriness in my eyes, and I have more energy." Her blood sugar levels were under control for the first time in years. And she did it all herself, mostly with dietary discipline.

Doctors seem to have changed too. They are pushing the self-responsibility part of health care. It used to be the doctors held some kind of magic knowledge, some special procedure or medicine that generates a cure. Now they advise patients on self-care as much as they provide treatment. They seem more open too, to alternative forms of medicine, to the role of attitude and motivation in healing.

The Internet has helped too. Now just about everyone in the United States has access to all kinds of in-depth medical knowledge, descriptions of medications, and educational resources for self-care and alternative medical treatments.

The big challenge now is overcoming the obstacles put in place by the need for corporate profits. There will always be a need for health care. Our knowledge is increasing daily, and the field of medicine needs well informed and motivated nurses.

* * *

Some of the developments I'm happy to see are the growing acceptance of ancillary and alternative forms of healing. This includes meditative practices, religious support, and spiritual insight.

Many health professionals have benefited from the research into death and dying, and the possibility of life after death. The International Association for Near-Death Studies (IANDS at www.iands.org) even offers a course on near-death experiences with continuing education credits (CEUs) for nurses.

* * *

Nursing is an excellent career choice for men and women alike. I hope, despite all the jokes and complaints, that you can appreciate the fantastic opportunity that nursing presents. It's a career that has meaning and value, and the better you do your job, the more people benefit. Directly.

Resources

Lists of Nursing Schools in America

- UnivSource:
  http://www.univsource.com/nurs.htm
- AllNursingSchools:
  http://www.allnursingschools.com/
- EdInformatics:
  http://www.edinformatics.com/nursing

Health Care Career Guides

- Vocational Information Center:
  http://www.khake.com/page22.html
- Lipincott's Nursing Center:
  http://www.nursingcenter.com/careerc
  enter/index.asp
- Guide to Health Care Schools:
  http://www.guidetohealthcareschools.
  com/careers/nurse

Nursing Organizations and Associations

- The Agape Center: http://www.theagapecenter.com/Organizations/Nursing.htm
- Nurse.org: http://www.nurse.org/orgs.shtml
- Discover Nursing: http://www.discovernursing.com/nursing-organizations

Helpful Sites

- American Nursing Association: http://www.nursingworld.org/
- American Assembly for Men in Nursing: http://www.aamn.org/
- All Nurses.com: http://allnurses.com/
- Nurse.com: http://www.nurse.com/
- NurseZone: http://www.nursezone.com/default.aspx

Information on Near-Death Experiences

- International Association for Near-Death Studies: http://www.iands.org
- Near-Death Experience Research Foundation: http://www.nderf.org
- Near-Death Experiences and the Afterlife: http://www.near-death.com/

Made in the USA
Lexington, KY
11 December 2011